CANNABIS

A practical guide for utilizing marijuana to enhance physical and mental state, enhance appearance, promote restful sleep, and improve overall wellness.

Oliver Wrench

1

Table of Contents

DISCLAIMER

This information is not intended to provide medical advice or substitute for the advice or treatment of a personal physician. It is suggested that you get counsel from your doctors or skilled health professionals regarding any particular health concerns you may have. Readers and followers of this educational resource are responsible for any potential health consequences.

Introduction

Oliver Wrench's captivating book "Cannabis" will introduce you to the world of cannabis and perhaps alter your perception of this amazing plant. Regardless of your interest in cannabis's medical properties, cultural effects, or prospective economic benefits, this book provides an in-depth, engrossing, and thorough investigation like no other.

Cannabis is a plant that is frequently entangled in controversy, but it is now coming out of the shadows, losing its stigma, and fulfilling its potential.

Travel back in time to when cannabis was a vital component of spiritual ceremonies and therapeutic rituals in ancient cultures. Learn how it was demonized and brought into disdain in the modern age, only for modern science and cultural movements to bring it back to life.

The exploration of cannabis's significant influence on

health and wellness is at the core of this book.

Cannabis shows up as a ray of hope in a society where mental health issues and chronic illnesses are rampant.

Examine the science of cannabinoids such as THC and CBD to learn how they work with our bodies to promote healing and comfort.

This book offers convincing facts that paint cannabis as a natural treatment ready to transform contemporary medicine, covering everything from anxiety to chronic pain.

The book "Cannabis" honors the plant's cultural and economic comeback in addition to its medical advantages. Examine the ways that cannabis is shattering barriers, changing norms, and impacting music, art, and social movements. Observe the economic explosion as innovation and cannabis farming provide employment and promote sustainable development. Cannabis is more than simply a plant; it is a force for good, a symbol of resiliency.

Join me in discovering its unseen narrative and imagining a future in which cannabis is valued for the numerous advantages it provides.

Start the path toward wellness now!

Chapter One

Introduction

The terms "cannabis," "weed," "pot," and "marijuana" all belong to a single botanical family renowned for their soothing and relaxing properties. However, the effects differ based on how you consume it, and it is prohibited in many areas.

The term "cannabis" describes the group that includes three psychoactive plants: Cannabis sativa, Cannabis indica, and Cannabis ruderalis. One of the most widely used medications in the world is produced when the flowers of these plants are collected and dried. Some refer to it as pot, some as weed, and several others as marijuana. The titles for cannabis are changing as it becomes legal in more places.

Cannabis is a phrase that is increasingly being used to refer to marijuana these days. Some believe that the name is more appropriate. Unlike terms like "weed" or "pot," which some associate with illicit usage, others perceive the name as more neutral.

In addition, the word "marijuana" is losing popularity because of its racial history. The main reasons people use cannabis are for its soothing and relaxing properties. It's also given in several US states to treat a variety of illnesses, such as glaucoma, chronic pain, and eating disorders. Remember that even though cannabis is derived from a plant and is regarded as natural, it may still have potent effects that can be both beneficial and harmful.

What exactly are the components of cannabis?

Over 120 various components, together referred to as

cannabinoids, make up cannabis. Experts are still unsure of how each cannabinoid works, but they do have a decent knowledge of two of them: cannabidiol (CBD) and tetrahydrocannabinol.

Each has its own unique uses and effects.

➤ **CBD:** Although this is a psychoactive cannabinoid, it doesn't make you feel intoxicated or euphoric, so you won't get "high." It's frequently used to lessen pain and inflammation. Additionally, it could lessen anxiety, seizures, migraines, and nausea. To the best of current knowledge, researchers are still working to determine the medicinal benefits of CBD.

➤ **THC:** This is the primary psychoactive ingredient in marijuana. The "high" that most people associate with cannabis is caused by THC.

Products made from cannabis might include either pure CBD, pure THC, or a mix of the two. However, the dried flower that most people identify as cannabis contains both cannabinoids, but some strains may contain significantly more of one than the other. Hemp has a lot of CBD but not any THC.

How does cannabis affect you in the short term?

There are several immediate impacts of cannabis use. While some are helpful, others raise additional red flags.

The following are among the most desirable immediate outcomes:

- Comfort
- Excitement
- You are experiencing the sights and sounds around you with greater intensity.
- Increased hunger

- Changed understanding of events and time

- Concentration and originality

In comparison to THC, these effects are frequently negligible in products with extremely high quantities of CBD.

However, some people may experience serious side effects from cannabis. Possible side effects include:

- Problems with coordination

- Delayed response time

- Nausea

- Drowsiness

- Fear

- Elevated heart rate

- Lower blood pressure

- Worry

Again, products with a higher CBD content than THC are less likely to cause these side effects.

Furthermore, the manner in which you consume cannabis can influence its immediate effects. The effects of cannabis smoking take impact quickly. If you consume cannabis orally, for example, through a pill or food, it can take a few hours before you experience any effects.

How does cannabis affect you in the long term?

Researchers are still working to completely comprehend cannabis use's long-term impacts. Numerous studies that have been conducted on this subject have only examined animals, and there is a great deal of contradictory data.

It will take much more extensive, long-term human research to completely comprehend the long-term impacts of cannabis use.

Cognitive development

A 2014 study emphasizes the possible effects of cannabis usage throughout adolescence on brain development.

This study shows that kids who begin using cannabis early in life typically experience greater memory and learning issues than teens who do not start using cannabis until later in life.

However, it's unknown how long-lasting these impacts are.

Teenagers who begin smoking cannabis may also be more vulnerable to mental health problems, such as schizophrenia, in the future. However, researchers are still unsure how strong this relationship is.

Reliance

Cannabis use can potentially lead to dependence in certain people. Some even report experiencing mood changes, irritability, and decreased appetite as withdrawal symptoms after they stop taking cannabis.

Those who begin using cannabis before the age of eighteen

have a four- to seven-fold higher risk of developing a cannabis use disorder than those who begin using it later in life, according to the National Institute on Drug Abuse.

Respiratory issues

The dangers associated with smoking cannabis are comparable to those associated with smoking tobacco. The airways' irritation and inflammation might be the cause of this. Cannabis may increase the chance of developing chronic obstructive pulmonary disease (COPD) and has been linked to bronchitis.

On the other hand, minimal evidence of a connection between cannabis usage and lung cancer has been found in recent research.

Is it legal to use cannabis?

While cannabis is still illegal in many locations, more and more regions are beginning to allow it for both medical and recreational use. For instance, some states in the US have legalized cannabis for both recreational and medical use. Some have limited its lawful usage to medicinal purposes.

However, cannabis is still prohibited by federal law in the US. The evidence for using CBD to treat pain and inflammation is encouraging.

It's commonly known that the prescription drug Epidiolex, which contains CBD, can lessen some types of seizures.

National regulations pertaining to cannabis also differ. While some consider any use of cannabis to be a serious felony, others allow the use of products that contain solely CBD. If you're interested in trying cannabis, you should first research the regulations in your location.

Chapter Two

Cannabis Species and Strains

Cannabis is a diverse genus with a wide range of species and strains, each with its own distinct properties and effects. Here's a thorough examination of the main species and noteworthy strains:

Cannabis Species

Cannabis sativa

Origin: Typically found in the equitorial regions of Africa, Central and South America, and Southeast Asia.

Mode: tall with slender, pale green leaves.

Growth: generally better suited for outdoor culture, with a longer flowering time.

Effects: Frequently linked to uplifting, energizing, and cerebral effects. Usually used during the day.

Cannabis indica

Origin: Indigenous to the Hindu Kush area, which encompasses portions of Pakistan, India, and Afghanistan.

Mode: shorter and bushier, with broad, dark-green leaves.

Growth: Suitable for indoor culture, with a shorter flowering period.

Effects: well-known for being soothing and having body-focused properties. It is typically utilized for relaxation purposes or during the evening hours.

Cannabis ruderalis

Origin: Russia and Central Europe are the places of origin.

Mode: hardy and small, with a rougher appearance.

Growth: It has a short growth cycle and auto-flowers, which depend on age rather than the light cycle.

Effects: Reduced THC concentration, often crossed with other species to create hybrids that bloom independently.

Cannabis Strains

Prior to exploring certain strains, it's crucial to understand that sativas' effects are somewhat broad. Not every individual will inevitably encounter all of these effects.

Each will react to strains in a unique way. Your endocannabinoid system, physiology, and tolerance to different cannabinoids are all distinct.

Your environment and past experiences will also affect how you feel.

- Are you with pals or total strangers?

- Has anything painful or traumatic recently happened?
- Is there something that you're anxious about that will happen in the next few days?

This kind of thing will affect how you feel about certain strains. For example, a long-time cannabis user with a high tolerance to THC may get an upbeat antidepressant effect from a high-THC sativa.

However, for someone with a lesser tolerance or who reacts differently to different terpene profiles, the experience can be extremely different.

Lastly, bear in mind that strains are not always uniform among brands and are by no means a precise science. If you enjoy a strain from one brand, you may notice that the same strain feels extremely different from another brand.

Energy Strains

Generally speaking, these strains are best used during the day to help with productivity and motivation.

- **Sour Diesel**

There's a good reason why this Chemdawg and Super Skunk hybrid is well-liked. Due to its increased THC content, seasoned cannabis users appear to return again and again to enjoy its stimulating effects, which may be beneficial for those suffering from depression. It contains 17–26% THC.

- **Jack Herer**

Another well-liked variety is called Jack Herer, after the novelist and cannabis activist. Reviews indicate that it is highly stimulating, and some users have said that it has helped with symptoms of depression. It contains 15–24% THC.

- **Green Crack**

Although the name of this strain may cause a bit of uncertainty, it is not that dissimilar from the strains mentioned above. It's a well-liked, widely accessible strain with stimulating properties. Similar to Jack Herer, a number of reviews claim feeling less depressed. It contains 15–25% THC.

Focus Strains

If you're looking for better focus, these strains could be worth a try.

- **Lucid Blue**

When it comes to concentration and attention, this hybrid of Blue Dream and Grateful Breath is highly recommended—that is, assuming you can find the strain, which could be more difficult than some others on the list. It contains 16–28% THC and 0–4% CBD.

- **Sour Breath**

This strain, which is a hybrid of Lamb's Bread and Sour Diesel, is well-known for its strong smell. Its ability to increase focus has received great reviews. If you're new to cannabis, this is an excellent pick because of its lower THC level. It contains 15–17% THC.

- **Red Congolese**

Red Congolese, another high-THC sativa, is becoming more well-known, partly because of its unique flavor, which has been characterized as fruity and cheesy.

Numerous reviews point out that it tends to provide focused clarity along with a little bit of physical relaxation. It contains 18–23% THC.

Creativity Strains

Want to break out of a slump or just explore your creative side? Consider these options.

- **Chocolope**

Compared to other of the heavier sativas on the list, chocolope often has a more moderate THC content, which results in slightly more relaxed effects. It contains 16–23% THC.

- **Super Silver Haze**

Super Silver Haze has a successful track record; in 1997, 1998, and 1999, it took home the first-place trophy at the High Times Cannabis Cup. It's also highly regarded for instilling a feeling of serenity and inspiring creativity. It contains 18–23% THC.

- **Durban Poison**

Many individuals consider this invigorating, pure sativa to be their go-to for stimulating creative thought. Many people report that it's the most stimulating strain they've ever experienced; it's the exact opposite of sedatives. It contains 17–26% THC.

Mood-Uplifting Strains

These strains can lift your spirits, whether you're feeling down or just want to feel nice.

- **Strawberry Cough**

One prevalent effect of Strawberry Cough, a sativa-dominant strain with an unknown origin, is happiness and exhilaration. It contains 17–23% THC.

- **Harlequin GDP**

If you're new to cannabis or have had anxiety-inducing encounters with cannabis sativa products in the past, this high-CBD strain is worth trying. It has a more mellow effect than many other sativas. It contains 3–7% CBD and 10–11% THC.

- **Super Lemon Haze**

Super Lemon Haze, another Cannabis Cup winner, is a hybrid of Lemon Skunk with the previously mentioned

Super Silver Haze. Many people who have used this strain have reported experiencing happiness, exhilaration, or both. It contains 18–25% THC.

Chapter Three

Chemical Composition

A family of chemical substances known as cannabinoids affects the release of neurotransmitters in the brain by binding to cannabinoid receptors in cells. The cannabis plant is where they are mostly found. Tetrahydrocannabinol (THC) and cannabidiol (CBD) are the two most well-known types of cannabinoids. The following is a quick summary of the main cannabinoids'

TETRAHYDROCANNABINOL (THC)

Chemical Formula: $C_{21}H_{30}O_2$

Structure: THC is a phenol group-containing bicyclic molecule. The terpenoid backbone of this substance aids in its solubility in fats and oils.

Psychoactivity: The primary psychoactive component of

cannabis, THC, is what gives users of cannabis the "high" they experience.

CANNABIDIOL (CBD)

Chemical Formula: $C_{21}H_{30}O_2$

Structure: The molecular structure of CBD is comparable to that of THC, while the atom arrangements are different. It is a hydroxyl group with a bicyclic molecule.

Psychoactivity: Cannabidiol (CBD) possesses no psychoactive effects and is well-known for its possible medicinal benefits, including its ability to reduce inflammation and anxiety.

CANNABINOL (CBN)

Chemical Formula: $C_{21}H_{26}O_2$

Structure: Degradation of THC yields CBN, a moderately psychoactive chemical. It has additional oxidation and a slightly different structure.

Psychoactivity: not as strong as THC.

CANNABIGEROL (CBG)

Chemical Formula: $C_{21}H_{32}O_2$

Structure: THC, CBD, and other cannabinoids are all derived from CBG, a non-psychoactive cannabinoid.

Psychoactivity: Non-psychoactive.

CANNABICHROMENE (CBC)

Chemical Formula: $C_{21}H_{30}O_2$

Structure: The molecular makeup of CBC is comparable to that of other cannabinoids, but it has a unique arrangement that adds to its own special set of effects.

Psychoactivity: Non-psychoactive.

CHEMICAL CHARACTERISTICS AND EFFECTS

LIPID SOLUBILITY: Cannabinoids can readily pass through blood-brain barriers and cell membranes because they are often lipid-soluble.

INTERACTION WITH RECEPTORS: As a component of the endocannabinoid system, cannabinoids mainly interact with CB1 and CB2 receptors. While CBD interacts with various receptor systems, it has a modest affinity for the CB1 receptors in the brain compared to THC's strong affinity for these receptors.

SYNTHESIS AND METABOLISM: The glandular trichomes of the cannabis plant are where cannabinoids are produced. They are converted by the liver into a variety of metabolites after intake or inhalation, some of which have pharmacological activity.

THERAPEUTIC AND RECREATIONAL

PURPOSES

THC: It is used medicinally and recreationally to relieve nausea, stiffness in the muscles, and pain. It also stimulates hunger.

CBD: It is widely utilized for treating chronic pain, anxiety, and epilepsy, among other conditions, for potential medicinal advantages without the psychoactive effects.

CBN, CBG, and CBC: They are being studied for their potential therapeutic benefits, which include anti-inflammatory, antibacterial, and neuroprotective properties.

Comprehending the molecular makeup and characteristics of cannabinoids is essential for the use of cannabis for medicinal and recreational purposes, as well as for the continuous investigation of its possible advantages and disadvantages.

Terpenes

Terpenes are an extensive and varied family of chemical

substances that are generated by a number of different plants, including cannabis. They may have medicinal benefits and are principally in charge of the flavor and fragrance of cannabis. The following are a few typical terpenes in cannabis:

Myrcene

Chemical Formula: $C_{10}H_{16}$

Structure: The monoterpene myrcene has a backbone of 10 carbons.

Properties: It smells earthy and musky and is well-known for its sedative properties.

Limonene

Chemical Formula: $C_{10}H_{16}$

Structure: The monocyclic monoterpene limonene has a backbone of 10 carbons.

Properties: It smells like citrus and is thought to have anti-anxiety and mood-enhancing properties.

Pinene

Chemical Formula: $C_{10}H_{16}$

Structure: Pinene is a bicyclic monoterpene.

Properties: It smells like pine and is well-known for its bronchodilator and anti-inflammatory properties.

Linalool

Chemical Formula: $C_{10}H_{18}O$

Structure: An acyclic monoterpene alcohol is linalool.

Properties: Known for its relaxing and anti-anxiety benefits, it has a flowery, lavender-like scent.

Caryophyllene

Chemical Formula: $C_{15}H_{24}$

Structure: Caryophyllene is classified as a bicyclic sesquiterpene.

Properties: It smells spicy and peppery and is well-known for its analgesic and anti-inflammatory qualities.

Flavonoids

Cannabis is one of the many plants that contain a varied class of phytonutrients known as flavonoids. They have a number of possible health advantages and add to the plant's taste, fragrance, and color.

Cannflavins

- **Cannflavin A**

Chemical Formula: $C_{21}H_{20}O_6$

Structure: Cannflavin A is a prenylated flavonoid.

Properties: Its anti-inflammatory qualities are well-known.

- **Cannflavin B**

Chemical Formula: $C_{21}H_{20}O_6$

Structure: The prenylation pattern is somewhat different but otherwise similar to Cannflavin A.

Properties: It shares anti-inflammatory properties with Cannflavin A.

Quercetin

Chemical Formula: $C_{15}H_{10}O_7$

Structure: Quercetin possesses a 3-hydroxyflavone backbone, making it a flavonol.

Properties: It possesses anti-inflammatory, anti-histamine, and antioxidant properties.

Apigenin

Chemical Formula: $C_{15}H_{10}O_5$

Structure: The fundamental flavonoid structure of apigenin distinguishes it as a flavone.

Properties: It possesses anxiolytic, antioxidant, and anti-inflammatory qualities.

Kaempferol

Chemical Formula: $C_{15}H_{10}O_6$

Structure: Another flavonol is kaempferol.

Properties: It contains anti-inflammatory, anti-cancer, and antioxidant qualities.

CHEMICAL CHARACTERISTICS AND EFFECTS

Terpenes and flavonoids have similar lipid solubility, which makes it easier for them to interact with cell membranes and increases their biological activity.

INTERACTION WITH RECEPTORS: Terpenes have the ability to modulate the effects of cannabinoids by interacting with both cannabinoid receptors and other brain receptors. Flavonoids frequently show their effects by inhibiting certain enzymes and having antioxidant properties.

SYNTHESIS AND METABOLISM: In plants, the phenylpropanoid pathway is used to synthesize flavonoids, whereas the mevalonate pathway is used to synthesize terpenes. These substances are processed by different body enzymes after consumption or administration, which adds to their pharmacological effects.

Understanding the structure and functions of terpenes and flavonoids is important for comprehending all of cannabis' medical uses as well as the entourage effect, which is when many of its parts work together to make the benefits stronger.

Chapter Four

Methods of Consumption: Advantages and Disadvantages

Marijuana, commonly known as cannabis, is a psychoactive substance produced from the cannabis plant. For thousands of years, it has been utilized for industrial, medical, and recreational uses.

There is a vast range of cannabis consumption techniques, each having advantages and disadvantages of its own.

Below is a summary of the most popular techniques:

Smoking

Methods: joints, blunts, pipes, and bongs

- **Advantages**

Rapid onset: Results are usually felt in a matter of minutes.

Control: Dosage may be easily controlled by stopping when the intended result is reached.

Availability: This is the most popular and extensively accessible approach.

- **Disadvantages**

Health risks: may result in respiratory problems and expose users to toxic fumes from burning fuel.

Odor: It emits a strong, distinct odor that is difficult to mask.

Short duration: The effects usually last between 1 and 3 hours.

Edibles

Methods: meals and drinks infused with cannabis

- **Advantages**

There is no need to inhale: there are no respiratory dangers.

Effects that last: Can provide relief for 4–8 hours.

Inconspicuous: This allows for consumption without drawing notice.

- **Disadvantages**

Delayed onset: It may take up to two hours to feel the effects, which might encourage excessive consumption.

Dosage control: risks of overconsumption due to difficulty in precisely dosing.

Digestive problems: Some people may experience stomach pain.

Vaping

Methods: vape pens, vaporizers

- **Advantages**

Healthier than smoking: It limits exposure to harmful combustion byproducts.

Inconspicuous: It generates a minimal smell and is easier to hide.

Rapid onset: Effects are felt within minutes.

- **Disadvantages**

Cost: Vaping accessories can be exorbitant.

Dependency on batteries: Equipment has to be maintained and charged.

Possible hazards: There are worries about the safety of vape liquids and components.

Tinctures

Methods: alcohol or oil-based cannabis extracts

- **Advantages**

Rapid onset: When taken sublingually, the effects start to show within 15 to 45 minutes (under the tongue).

Convenient and discrete: simple to use and carry without creating any notice.

Accurate dosing: simpler to regulate and quantify dosages.

- **Disadvantages**

Flavor: Some people may find the flavor unpleasant.

Cost: Compared to alternative methods, this approach might be more expensive.

Topicals

Methods: creams, salves, lotions

- **Advantages**

Localized relief: useful for reducing pain or inflammation in certain regions.

Absence of psychoactive effects: not a high producer, therefore it's good for non-recreational usage.

Simple to utilize: straightforward skin application.

- **Disadvantages**

Restricted effects: does not relieve systemic symptoms; primarily helpful for localized ones.

Differential absorption: Depending on the product and the person, effectiveness may differ.

Capsules and Pills

Methods: Ingestible cannabis capsules

- **Advantages**

There are no respiratory hazards: it prevents breathing in mist or smoke.

Easy to use and concealed: simple to transport and ingest.

Accurate dosing: precise and accurate dosage.

- **Disadvantages**

Delay in onset: Effects might take 30 minutes to 2 hours to manifest.

Gastrointestinal problems: possible pain in the stomach.

Dabbing

Methods: Breathing in vapor from cannabis concentrates.

- **Advantages**

High effects: Delivers a powerful, short-lived high. Rapid onset: impact is perceived nearly instantly.

Efficiency: Minimal amounts are required to have a big impact.

- **Disadvantages**

Health risks: Dangerous chemicals can still be produced at high temperatures.

Complexity: This may be difficult for novices and requires specialized equipment.

Strong effects: For inexperienced users, this may be too much.

Users must select the cannabis ingestion technique that best suits their needs, lifestyle, and health considerations because each approach has certain advantages and disadvantages.

Chapter Five

Medical and Recreational Use of Cannabis

Cannabis usage has been increasingly popular in recent years, both for medicinal and recreational uses. Here's a summary of its medicinal applications, advantages, hazards, and status for recreational use:

Medical Usage of Cannabis

APPLICATIONS:

- **Chronic Pain Management:** Cannabis is frequently used to treat chronic pain, particularly in diseases like multiple sclerosis and arthritis.

- **Mental Health:** Although its effectiveness varies, it is occasionally used to treat depression, PTSD, and anxiety.

- **Cancer:** Pain, nausea, and appetite loss are just a few of the symptoms that cannabis can assist with.

- **Neurodegenerative Diseases:** Research indicates that people suffering from Parkinson's and Alzheimer's disease may benefit from cannabis use.

- **Epilepsy:** A few cannabis-derived medications, including Epidiolex, are licensed to treat severe and uncommon types of epilepsy.

The benefits include:

- **Pain Relief:** When other treatments have not worked, this method is helpful for many individuals with persistent pain.

- **Appetite Stimulation:** It helps patients who have lost their appetite due to conditions like HIV/AIDS or cancer treatments.

- **Anti-inflammatory:** The anti-inflammatory qualities of cannabinoids can aid in the treatment of a number of inflammatory diseases.

Hazards and adverse reactions:

- **Cognitive Impairment:** Extended use may cause memory loss and other cognitive impairments.

- **Mental Health Disorders:** Cannabis may occasionally make mental health disorders like paranoia and anxiety worse.

- **Abuse and Dependency:** Dependency is a possibility, particularly with strains that are THC-dominant.

Cannabis Usage for Recreation

Legalization and Status

- **Global Variance:** Cannabis laws pertaining to recreational use differ greatly. Some nations have decriminalized its usage, but others, like Uruguay and Canada, have completely legalized it.

- **United States:** Although it is still banned federally, recreational cannabis is allowed in a number of states, including California, Colorado, and Washington.

The benefits include:

- **Social and Recreational Enjoyment:** Many users report that cannabis improves social interactions and relaxation.

- **Economic Impact:** Legal cannabis markets provide jobs, increase tax income, and lower law enforcement expenses.

HAZARDS:

- **Health Concerns:** Smoking cannabis can provide respiratory hazards comparable to those associated with tobacco use.

- **Impaired Driving:** Cannabis usage can slow down response times and impair motor abilities, which raises the risk of accidents.

- **Impact on Youth:** Adolescents' early and extensive usage might interfere with brain development and cause cognitive problems.

Cannabis has been shown to have significant medicinal advantages, particularly in the treatment of chronic pain and other diseases. But there are hazards associated with using it, including possible dependency and cognitive effects.

Many areas are beginning to permit recreational usage more and more, and the main forces behind this trend are social and economic rewards. To ensure appropriate and informed usage, it is crucial to weigh these advantages against the hazards to one's health and safety.

Health Effects of cannabis: Short-term, long-term, psychological impact and physical health concerns

There are a number of short- and long-term psychological and physical health impacts of cannabis use.

SHORT-TERM HEALTH EFFECTS

Psychological Impact:

- *Relaxation and Euphoria:* Cannabis frequently results in emotions of relaxation, euphoria, and altered time perception.

- *Impaired Attention and Memory:* There can be major impairments to attention and memory in the short term.

- *Psychomotor Impairment:* Cannabis impairs motor abilities, response times, and coordination, which raises the possibility of mishaps.

- *Anxiety and Paranoia:* When using strong THC strains, some users may have increased anxiety, paranoia, or panic attacks.

Physical Health Issues:

- *Dryness of the mouth and eyes:* Users frequently report dry mouths (cottonmouth) and dry, red eyes.

- *Elevated Heart Rate:* Using cannabis may result in a brief elevation in heart rate.

- *Appetite Stimulation:* Cannabis, which is frequently seen as "the munchies," has the potential to enhance appetite.

- *Respiratory Issues:* The lungs may become irritated as a result of smoking cannabis, resulting in symptoms similar to bronchitis and severe coughing.

LONG-TERM HEALTH EFFECTS

Psychological Impact:

- *Mental Health Disorders:* Long-term use is associated with an elevated risk of mental health disorders, including depression, anxiety, and, in certain instances, psychosis and schizophrenia, particularly in individuals who are predisposed to these conditions.
- *Cognitive Decline:* The reduction of IQ and cognitive decline can result from the chronic, heavy use of cannabis, particularly during adolescence.

- *Addiction and Dependency:* Approximately 9% of cannabis users may have addiction and dependency as a result of cannabis use disorder.

Physical Health Issues:

- *Respiratory Issues:* Chronic cannabis smoking can result in respiratory problems that are comparable to those caused by tobacco smoking, such as chronic bronchitis and lung infections.

- *Suppression of the Immune System:* According to certain research, long-term cannabis usage may weaken the immune system, leaving the body more vulnerable to diseases.

- *Cardiovascular Problems:* Extended usage may raise the risk of heart disease and stroke, especially in people with underlying medical disorders.

ACKNOWLEDGEMENTS

God alone is worthy of all praise. In addition, I would like to express my gratitude to my amazing family, partner, readers, fans, friends, and customers for their unwavering encouragement and support.

www.ingramcontent.com/pod-product-compliance
Lightning Source LLC
Chambersburg PA
CBHW031135020426
42333CB00012B/389